Bread Machine Cookbook

An assortment of delicious and fragrant recipes, for making your own bread at home

DEAN LOXLEY

Table of Contents

INTRODUCTION 10

CONFIGURATION OF A BREAD MACHINE 11

CRITERIA FOR SELECTING THE RIGHT BREAD MACHINE 12

HOW MUCH DO YOU WISH TO BAKE BREAD? 13

HOW MUCH WILL YOU USE THE GADGET TO MAKE BREAD? 13

CAN YOU SAVE TIME, WITH A BREAD MACHINE? 14

WHAT IS THE EXPENSE OF THE BREAD MAKING MACHINE? 15

ARE YOU PLANNING ON ENTERTAINING WITH FRIENDS AND

FAMILY? 15

WILL YOU TRY NEW FOODS? 16

IS THE COMPACTED DENSE BREAD JUST AS GOOD? 17

HOW DOES THE BREAD MACHINE WORK? 18

WHY SHOULD YOU CONSIDER BUYING A BREAD MACHINE? 19

Tidy, Convenient, and Smooth to Run 19

The Healthy Range 20

WHEN YOU'RE UNFAMILIAR WITH THE BAKING OF BREAD 21

ADVANTAGES OF BREAD MACHINE 21

CERTAIN DISADVANTAGES OF BREAD MACHINE 25

CHAPTER 1. BREAKFAST RECIPES 27

CHERRY-PECAN COCOA BREAD 28

HONEY BUTTERMILK BREAD 29

OATMEAL BREAD WITH MOLASSES AND HONEY 31

SWEETENED CONDENSED MILK WHITE BREAD 32

MOLASSES WHEAT BREAD 34

CRUSTY BREAD MACHINE ROLLS 35

CRUSTY FRENCH BREAD 37

WHEAT BERRY BREAD 39

DARK RYE BREAD...42

SOFT GIANT PRETZELS 43

PUMPKIN MONKEY BREAD..45

BLUEBERRY ROLLS 48

GRUYÈRE APPLE PIE CINNAMON BUNS WITH VANILLA MOCHA

GLAZE...50

CHAPTER 2. LUNCH RECIPES 54

FLAVORFUL HERB BREAD 55

PEPPERONI PIZZA..56

HERBED PESTO BREAD 58

WHOLE WHEAT PIZZA DOUGH WITH HONEY............................59

MINI MAPLE CINNAMON ROLLS.. 61

PUMPKIN QUICK BREAD 63

ALL STEAK ORANGE ROLLS...65

BRAIDED ONION-POTATO LOAF 68

CALZONE ROLLS..70

ONION FRENCH BREAD LOAVES 72

GARLIC HERB BUBBLE LOAF 74

CIABATTA BREAD 76

WHEAT BERRY BREAD..78

CHAPTER 3. DINNER RECIPES 81

HAMBURGER BUNS 82

JEWISH CHALLAH 84

MEAT PIZZA DOUGH 86

GARLIC PIZZA DOUGH 88

KALAMATA OLIVE BREAD 90

WHOLE WHEAT CRESCENT DINNER ROLLS 92

ROSE ROLLS WITH ROSE BUTTERCREAM 94

SUN-DRIED TOMATO AND OLIVE LOAF 97

HAWAIIAN DINNER ROLLS 99

MEAT PIZZA DOUGH 101

QUICK AND SOFT DINNER ROLLS 103

SOUR CREAM CHIA BREAD 105

CAJUN BREAD..106

CHAPTER 4. DESSERT RECIPES 109

SWEET BANANA BREAD WITH YEAST.. 110

CRANBERRY SAUCE ROLLS 113

BREAD BEAR CLAWS 115

CINNAMON ROLL USING THE TANGZHONG 118

BASIC CINNAMON ROLLS.. 121

BLUEBERRY ROLLS 124

GLAZED YEAST DOUGHNUTS 127

CHOCOLATE BREAD 129

FROSTED CINNAMON ROLLS.. 133

CHOCOLATE CHIP PEANUT BUTTER BANANA BREAD 135

APPLE KUCHEN 137

ENGLISH MUFFIN BREAD 140

CHERRY 'N CHEESE LATTICE COFFEE CAKE 142

CONCLUSION **145**

Introduction

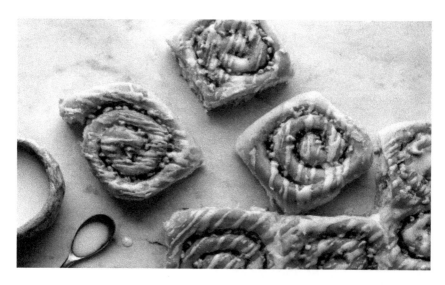

A bread machine is a kitchen appliance for converting raw materials into baked bread. It includes a bread pan, one or more designed paddles at the base of which are placed in the middle of a tiny, particularly unique oven. Typically, this little oven is operated by a standard built-in device through a control panel using the settings input.

Many even have a timer to enable the bread machine's activation without the operator's attendance, and some high-end versions allow the consumer to plan a custom period.

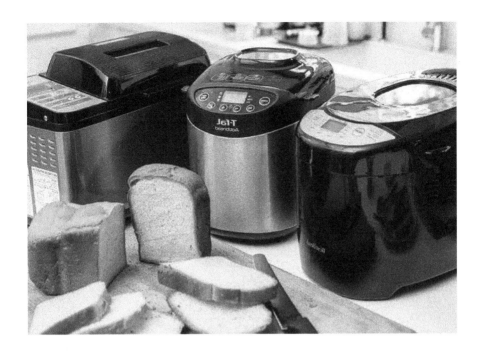

Configuration of a Bread Machine

The bread maker is made up of many elements. This machine is a small electric oven holding a single, wide bread tin inside. It has an adapter at the bottom that is attached to an electric motor beneath. The container itself is a little unusual.

At the bottom of the tin, a flat metal paddle is fixed to the axle. The paddle is liable for the dough being kneaded. A watertight lock protects the axle itself.

Let's look in-depth at each of the pieces of the bread machine:

The lid on top of the bread machine comes either with or without the display pane.

For ease, the control panel is often placed on the top of the bread machine.

There is a steam vent in the middle of the lid that exhausts the steam throughout the baking process. On the device side, some of the bread makers often have an air vent to come into the tin for the dough to rise.

Criteria for Selecting the Right Bread Machine

Think of yourself what the criteria will be before selecting the right kind of bread machine for yourself.

- **Timer:** You can manually determine when to set the timer for a baking cycle. Then you have to come at the right time, to take the bread out of the maker. Otherwise, the bread would be preheated and cooked, or choose a one where the machine will calculate the time.

- **Size:** Get the bread machine that carries a recipe comprising 3 cups of flour if one has a big family. Some can hold flour cups of up to 4 to 5 and a half.

- **Blades:** Blades in horizontal pans do not often knead the dough too well, leaving the pan's corners with flour. A significant negative is incomplete blending. However, the upright settings do a better job of mixing. Many new machines are made vertically, but some horizontal pans also offer two blades, so choose carefully.

How Much Do You Wish to Bake Bread?

Purchasing the bread machine makes perfect sense if you bake daily. The appliance must have been combining and kneading the dough properly that makes things easy for you. Using a bread machine will save you a lot of time and effort as it will make you knead the dough without too much trouble.

How Much Will You Use the Gadget to Make Bread?

Besides, ask yourselves how much you intend the bread machine to be used for bread baking. Are you or your friends mindful with your food, and can you want bread that is vegan or gluten-free? If so, purchasing a bread machine will save you a lot of money compared to purchasing organic bread in a store. The chances are that the bread machine will be regularly utilized if you bake at least once a week.

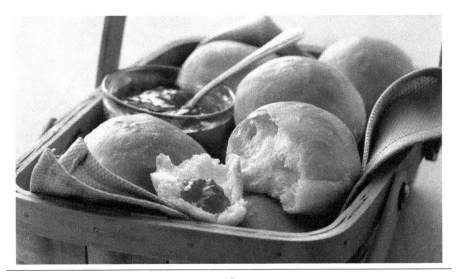

Can You Save Time, With a Bread Machine?

We live busy lives. With a bread machine, baking bread will be easy. Without it, you have to add the spices that need to be applied, knead the dough, allow it to rise for a bit, and finally bake the bread. It is a long tiresome procedure.

Bread normally requires about four hours to produce. If you can spare a little time, why not complete this task?

While oven baking bread is an automatic operation, the bread is kneaded by hand in a manual baker. For the robots, you can place the ingredients you want, retrieve what is needed, and then put it into the oven to bake at the correct time. This bread maker's best feature is its capacity to bake bread in much less than an hour. Even though bread machines are tactile, you should consult their characteristics to determine which to buy as a consequence of your lifestyle.

What Is the Expense of the Bread Making Machine?

One of the most critical aspects to often decide by looking at bread machines' reports is the price point. Any reasonably cheap but good quality bread makers last long time periods, offering one incredible value. An affordable bread maker is a safer option than the more costly and accurate model for occasional baking. If you are going to make bread daily, on the other side, you need a better model, including the Zojirushi BB-PCD20BA or the CBK 200 2Lb Bread Maker. In the future, I believe buying these high-quality bread machines would have a really good return for your capital.

Are You Planning on Entertaining With Friends and Family?

As a social practice, would you like to impress your peers while they enter your home? Help them feel comfortable by surprising them with freshly baked bread. Many of the elders in our community used to make bread. Get one of those modern bread-making devices if your buddies and relatives usually drop by. You may not be able to make fresh bread for your family with this appliance, but you will still be able to save on the expense of buying bread every day. Get your hands on one of the best bread-making devices if you have a big family.

Will You Try New Foods?

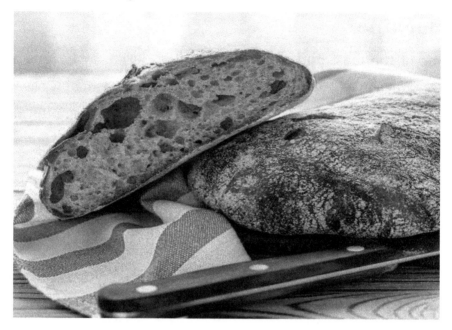

If you're a bread maker (or you used to be), you'll want to learn how you can make something new for yourself when you buy a Bread Machine. If you have some curiosity about Japanese cuisine, the Panasonic SD-BMS105-SW is suggested. This bread machine can create various items, such as

a melon pan, a red bean bread, a brioche, a steamed bun, a mochi, and several more. There are many online recipes for bread with quirky results. You may even produce bread with your bread machine.

Is the Compacted Dense Bread Just as Good?

Yeah, since it is made from the same ingredients and could be easier in certain situations, you may create different ingredients for your bread and use your whole grains. In reality, some people prefer bread from the bread machine to store-bought loaves or oven-baked. For a thickly textured toast, there's plenty to be told. On the other side, a piece of bread is so much better if it has risen better, is lighter in color, and fluffier.

Both the styles of bread seen in the picture were produced from the same recipe. They began in the bread maker, one on a single rotation that included baking mostly in the machine (tall loaf), while one was made on the dough setting and baked in a range of ovens (horizontal loaf). The normal heavier texture of the machine bread, while the oven-baked loaf grew higher and lighter. Sunbeam was the bread maker that was used in this research.

How does the Bread Machine Work?

In the same direction indicated and the period selected, recipe ingredients are inserted into the machine's bread pan. The bread dough would be combined and kneaded by the machine, taken through a rest time and first lifted, then raised to the second and ended by baking the bread in the machine. Complete intervals can vary from 2 to 3 hours; there are countdown timers on several equipment types.

After the shorter step is done (first rising), devices with a dough setting allow you to detach the bread dough where you can then mold it manually, which will enable it to rise and finish the baking bread phase in your oven range.

Why Should You Consider Buying a Bread Machine?

Whenever you need to prepare loads of loaves or need extra comfort, you can get a bread machine. You may be tired of hand-making bread and have a full life or any sort of disability. Bread machines are quite easy, convenient, and worth any cent at the end of the day.

In bread baking, kneading is probably the most difficult physical effort. Yeah, I like the dough's sensation on my hands, but for different purposes, whether it be health reasons, the exhaustion that comes with age, or some other excuse you might think of, many people do not have the stamina.

A bread machine is a perfect solution for anyone who wants to "get around" this move. It immediately kneads the dough and does an amazing job at it. So, even though you want to do anything yourself, the kneading portion may surely be given to the bread machine's capable hands.

Tidy, Convenient, and Smooth to Run

Baking bread is a thousand-year-old ancient art that involves us and our kitchen to give ourselves to crafts. We find ourselves spending our time washing the kitchen, the flour and bits of dough off the counter, the dishes in the wash, all that jazz, rather than sitting and waiting silently for the bread to come out of the oven, instead of focusing on the dough.

The entire thing is rendered so much simpler by the bread machine.

Put the ingredients in the bread maker, push a lever, set the timer, and that's all you have to do. The kitchen remains tidy, and waiting for the bread to be ready is all that's left to do.

This consideration becomes critical if you bake bread regularly and despite the rigorous routine that most of us maintain and know so well.

Timing: a bread machine would have built-in times to avoid mixing, make a rise, punch out the bread, and so on, unlike a mixer. Machines will bake bread as well, clearly, but mixers can't.

The Healthy Range

Like someone who produces his bread, it's a much better choice to make bread at home than purchasing bread at a bakery or even certain delicatessens, in which most bread is produced with a certain degree of improvement in baking.

You should select better foods when choosing which products to use in your food, whether it's organic grain, gluten-free bread, whole wheat, or whatever your food restrictions or preferences are.

There is a wide range of cookbooks built specifically for bread machines to help you obtain your bread gold on the market. To learn all about this, click here right now.

When You're Unfamiliar With the Baking of Bread

If you don't have the time to study and have little practice, you also want freshly baked bread. The bread machine can turn you into a professional baker. You can save cash, save energy (you know what you put in your body), and eat fresh bread.

Advantages of Bread Machine

When making your organic bread, you can monitor the ingredients used to make it. As I mentioned, you can combine components such as oats or quinoa or flax seeds, or something. You may opt to use sugar-free flour and even determine whether you like extra or less sweet. You can often add less salt in homemade bread on some loaves of bread/biscuits instead of shop purchases.

By utilizing a hundred percent whole-grain wheat flour and some other of the whole grain's flour, you will produce nutritious bread. When it comes to fiber and nutrients, whole grain helps the body to get more of both.

Many people mix extra flour into their bread to produce pasta. Others substitute the trans fats with olive oil. A final problem is the shortage of sodium (unless you add vegetable shortening or margarine). To keep the bread lasting longer, it would be set out of the freezers. This gives more taste, which will not go bad without the preservatives and additives.

While bread that is usually purchased in the supermarket produces about 13 g of sodium per 100 g (two to three slices), it is a rather small volume. Far under the recommended daily quantity of 6 g/day, you are in control of what flavors are included for what proteins when you prepare your own meals from scratch, whether it's with low-sodium salt or some other well-balanced option, such as herbs, spices, or pepper.

If you look at the ingredients in a bag of your favorite bread, you can have a hard time understanding what a product is, particularly if it is slightly fresh. Homemade bread doesn't contain any ingredients. These condiments, emulsifiers, exotic ingredients, and preservatives make it possible for the cake to obtain a longer shelf life, and so it is also simpler to prepare.

Bake your own and simply use the same ingredients as mentioned in the recipe and play with a variety of different flours, including rye or spelt. What it means is that if you're baking cookies, producing sandwiches, or roasting your nuts, you can quickly tailor your approach to your favorite location. Everyone's dietary needs can be accommodated without checking the shelves for an expensive expert loaf, whether or not they choose to eat more fiber or whether they would like to take out gluten. And if you don't have time to weigh and knead the bread yourself, like most of us do, simply inject the ingredients into a bowl and encourage the bread machine to do all the hard work for you. The fat can be lost without wasting the loaf. The finest bread in the store is still not as cholesterols as it was once before.

If you are trying to bake your bread, you might swap the usual white bread you usually purchase for a better option, like whole grain, or use a heart-healthy oil like olive oil. Positive news, that it means you're working desperately to shed weight. You also feel the same towards your food to include bread. You take this to encourage dietary change.

Bringing in several seeds will not be simple, but baking bread into a meal instead places the seeds in a sneaky position with not even the host to note. Consider introducing loaves of bread with these ingredients to your dietary menu: calcium, which gives the bread its taste and shape; linseed, which adds strength and moisture; healthy fats to create a brown color; sesame seeds, which offer you more substance, and lentils for more protein.

To stop conflicting effects if you have an extreme reaction to such things, change the recipes, so they do not contain certain allergenic ingredients.

Due to the chemical interactions in a bread's ingredients, many of your baked bread components can be selected and picked by you. Be sure you use the cheapest, freshest ingredients, like rice, milk, and dairy goods. Milk and juice are still regulated, so you don't have to worry about the possibility that your cereal includes "high fructose corn syrup" or "dextrose" and has a little health benefit.

As compared to industrial, mass-produced loaves of bread, homemade bread does not contain trans fats because you replace the butter or shortening in your recipe. It would help if you instead used unsaturated fats like olive oil or safflower oil. To extend their shelf life and boost taste, commercially baked bread often contains preservatives and chemical additives, while homemade bread does not.

Certain Disadvantages of Bread Machine

The machine's paddle often gets stuck in the bread, and when it is removed, a hole is caused at the end of the bread, which is a nightmare for trying to make sandwiches.

Some machines are limited to their pre-set program.

Bread makers can be fiddly to clean.

They use a lot of electricity.

Most bread makers last for a limited number of loaves.

Chapter 1. Breakfast Recipes

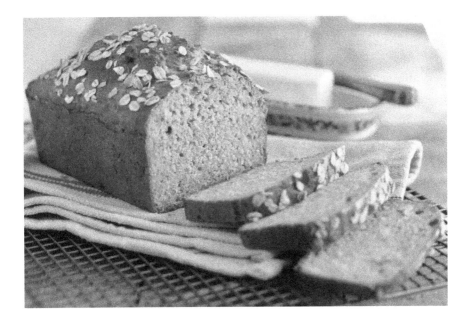

Cherry-Pecan Cocoa Bread

Preparation Time: 3 hours 10 minutes |Servings: 16 slices |Difficulty: Medium

Ingredients:

- Water (room temperature)1/3 cup
- Chopped pecans, half cup
- Dried cherries, half cup
- Butter softened, five tablespoons
- Salt one teaspoon
- Bread flour, three cups
- Baking cocoa, five tablespoons
- Packed brown sugar, 1/3 cup
- Warm whole milk (room temperature)2/3 cup
- Active dry yeast, two and a quarter teaspoon

Instructions:

1. In the bread machine pan, place the ingredients in the order proposed by the maker.

2. Pick the simple setting for the bread. If available, choose the crust color and loaf size.

3. After 5 minutes of mixing, check the dough; add one to two tablespoons of water or flour as needed. Apply the pecans and cherries just before the last kneading (your bread machine can audibly signal this).

4. Bake according to the instructions.

Honey Buttermilk Bread

Preparation Time:3 hours 10 minutes |Servings:4 |Difficulty: Medium

Ingredients:

- Water half cup

- Bread flour, three cups

- Salt, one and a half teaspoon

- Yeast, two teaspoons

- Buttermilk (well shaken) 3/4 cup

- Honey, three-tablespoon

- Butter (softened) three teaspoons.

- Garnish; poppy seeds, caraway seeds, or sesame seeds.

- Egg wash; egg white one large and two teaspoons water

Instructions:

1. Collect all the ingredients.

2. Place all the ingredients in the order proposed by the maker of the bread machine. Choose a simple or white bread environment and a light or medium crust.

3. Use the cycle of the dough to mold the bread into a sandwich.

4. Place the loaf with one large white egg and two teaspoons of water on an oiled sheet or in a pan and apply egg wash. Sprinkle the bread with sesame seeds if needed.

5. Bake for around 30 minutes at 375° F.

6. Enjoy and serve.

Oatmeal Bread with Molasses and Honey

Preparation Time: 3 hours 10 minutes |Servings:8 |Difficulty: Medium

Ingredients:

- Water (boiling) one cup

- Yeast (sprinkled over flour) two teaspoons.

- Honey, three-tablespoon

- One large egg (lightly beaten)

- Dark molasses, one tablespoon

- Butter, two tablespoons

- Salt, one and a half teaspoon

- Oats (old-fashioned) half cup

- Bread flour, three cups

Instructions:

1. In a mixing container, place the oats. Over the oats, add one cup of hot water, and set aside.

2. Move them to the pan if the oats have cooled and are also a little warmer (about 105° F to 110° F).

3. According to the manual of your bread machine maker, put the rest of the ingredients.

4. The recipe creates a loaf of one and a half pounds.

Sweetened Condensed Milk White Bread

Preparation Time: 3 hours 30 minutes |Servings:4 |Difficulty: Hard

Ingredients:

- Water (room temperature) 8 ounces

- Instant yeast, two scant teaspoons

- Bread flour (360 grams) three cups

- Salt, one teaspoon

- Sweetened condensed milk, half cup

- Butter (room temperature) one tablespoon

Instructions:

1. Place all ingredients in the bread pan.

2. Click and start the Dough cycle.

3. Lift the lid and, after around 10 minutes, check the dough. If required, apply the flour one tablespoon at a time until the dough hits the desired consistency. It can fall together in a ball that gathers cleanly to the surface of the pan and then pulls away. If the dough thumps against the bowl's surface, apply one tablespoon of warm water at a time. Add flour one tablespoon before the dough tends to shape a mild softball if the dough is sticky and doesn't break away from the hand.

4. Lift the dough from the pan and put it on a lightly floured plank. To pressure out some big air bubbles, knead a little bit by side.

5. Roll about 9 x 11 inches into a rectangle. Starting from the long end, roll up and tuck the ends to fit into the 9 x 4-inch oiled loaf sheet. Let it increase until the original size of the dough is doubled. Since this dough is a "high-riser," be cautious not to let the dough rise too much because it may cave in on the sides and the top.

6. Preheat the oven for 15 minutes before predicting that your loaf would be finished.

7. Bake for 35-45 minutes at 375°F. The interior is predicted to exceed 190°F. Place a foil over the bread halfway through baking to guard against over-browning.

8. Let it sit 15 minutes to cool. It's better to wait at least 2 hours before slicing so that the loaf maintains its form under the weight of a knife without squishing.

Molasses Wheat Bread

Preparation Time: 4 hours 10 minutes |Servings: One loaf |Difficulty: Hard

Ingredients:

- One and 3⁄4 cups, Whole wheat flour

- 3/4 cup of water

- Three tablespoons of melted butter

- 1⁄3 cup of milk

- Two tablespoons of sugar

- Three tablespoons of molasses

- Two and a quarter teaspoon of fast-rising yeast

- Two cups of bread flour

- One teaspoon of salt

Instructions:

1. Add all the ingredients to the machine according to your suggested machine's order. Make sure the ingredients are at room temperature

2. Use light crust, basic setting.

3. Serve fresh.

Crusty Bread Machine Rolls

Preparation Time:2 hours 30 minutes |Servings:8 |Difficulty: Hard

Ingredients:

- Water, one cup

- Salt, one and a half teaspoon

- Olive oil, one tablespoon

- Sugar, one and a half teaspoon

- Bread flour, one and a half cup

- All-purpose unbleached flour, one and a half cup

- Bread machine or instant yeast, one teaspoon

Glaze:

- A quarter cup water plus half teaspoon cornstarch mixed in two cups and heated in a microwave for 20 seconds.

Instructions:

1. Heat one cup of tap water in a microwave for a minute. With the blade in place, put it into the bread machine pan.

2. Use the pan to combine olive oil, salt, sugar, rice, and yeast. Pick the cycle for the dough. Check the dough after 5 minutes. It can stick and draw away from the hand. If the dough is too wet, apply one tablespoon of starch, or add one

tablespoon of water at the time the dough is a little too soft (dough slaps against the side).

3. If the yeast period is over and the bread has increased to twice the initial amount, remove the dough on a floured surface.

4. Break the dough in half for dinner rolls, then cut each half in half (4 bits) and then divide every one of those pieces in half again, resulting in eight rolls. Shape yourself into balls.

Crusty French Bread

Preparation Time: 3 hours 40 minutes |Servings: One loaf |Difficulty: Hard

Ingredients:

- One teaspoon of instant yeast

- One and a half teaspoons of sugar

- One cup of lukewarm water

- One and a half teaspoons salt

- One and a half teaspoons of butter

- Three cups of bread flour

Glaze:

- One teaspoon of water

- One egg white

Instructions:

1. Add all the ingredients required to the bread machine as per your machine's suggested order.

2. Select the dough cycle. Adjust the dough's consistency after 5 to 10 minutes by adding one tablespoon of water at a time for very dry dough or one tablespoon of flour if it's too sticky. It should pull away after sticking to the sides.

3. When the machine beeps and the dough is done, take it out on a clean, floured surface. Shape into cylinder shape loaves. Shape into French bread.

4. Place the loaves in oiled baking pans. Cover with a towel and let it rise in a warm place.

5. Let the oven preheat to 425° F.

6. Make the glaze by mixing water with egg.

7. Coat the loaf's surface with a glaze.

8. Make cuts onto the dough surface.

9. Bake in the oven for 20 minutes.

10. Lower the oven's temperature to 350° F, bake for 5 to 10 minutes more or until golden brown.

11. Check the bread's internal temperature. It should be 195° F.

12. Cool slightly and serve fresh.

Wheat Berry Bread

Preparation and Bake Time: 4 hours |Servings:4 |Difficulty: Hard

Ingredients:

- Whole-grain wheat berries, half-cup (160 gr)

- Bread flour divided (300 grams) two and a half cups.

- Warm milk (or whey drained from yogurt) one cup (240 gr)

- Table salt, one and a half (6 gr) teaspoon

- Sugar, one teaspoon (4 gr)

- Unsalted butter softened, two tablespoons (28 gr)

- Bread machine or instant yeast, two teaspoons (6 gr)

Instructions:

1. Boil the wheat berries for 20 minutes in one cup of water. Let it cool (more easily if ice cubes are added) and drain. Alternatively, for 12 hours or overnight, boil the wheat berries in water.

2. Add prepared wheat berries with one cup of bread flour to a blender or food processor (120 grams). Process until you have finely chopped wheat berries. To transfer the flour and wheat berries from all the sides of the container back to the middle, you would need to pause many times.

3. Combine the milk or whey, the salt, the sugar, the butter, the remaining 180 grams of flour, the combination of ground-wheat-beer-and-flour, and the yeast.

4. Pick the cycle for the dough and begin. After 10 minutes, inspect the dough and ensure that the dough sticks to the pan's surface and then pulls away neatly. If it is too wet, apply one tablespoon more flour at a time. If it's too dusty, use one tablespoon more water at a time.

5. Check that the dough has increased in size (almost doubled) after the dough cycle ends. If not, hold it in the pan until it's finished.

6. Lift the dough from the pan to the floured surface and cut into two separate parts when doubled. Pull dough from top to bottom until dough is smooth, form each piece into an oblong shape; then pinch closed on a baking sheet filled with a silicone mat that's been coated with a touch of cornmeal, put seam side down.

7. Cover and let it rise until almost doubled with a tea towel. Preheat the oven to 425 °F for about 20 minutes until the loaf is ready to roast.

8. Apply loaves with one egg white glaze whipped with one tablespoon of sugar.

9. Using a razor blade or a sharp knife to create two-three diagonal slashes in each loaf, taking note not to deflate the dough.

10. Bake for 20 to 25 minutes in a preheated oven, or until the inside temperature is 190° F, or until the bottom is brown and sounds hollow.

11. Let the loaves be cool for an hour on a rack before slicing.

Dark Rye Bread

Preparation Time: 3 hours 10 minutes |Servings: One loaf |Difficulty: Hard

Ingredients:

- One and a quarter cups of warm water

- Two and a quarter teaspoon of Yeast

- One cup of rye flour

- Two and a half cups of bread flour

- 1/3 cup of molasses

- Half teaspoon of salt

- One tablespoon of Caraway seed

- 1/8 cup of Vegetable oil

- 1/8 cup of Cocoa powder

Instructions:

1. Place all the ingredients in the machine in the suggested order by the manufacturer.

2. Select white bread—Press the start button.

3. Serve fresh.

Soft Giant Pretzels

Preparation **Time:** **20** **min** **|Servings:8** **|Difficulty: Easy**

Ingredients:

- Water (room temperature), divided one cup plus two tablespoons

- Baking soda, half cup

- Water, two quarts

- Coarse salt

- Active dry yeast, one and a half teaspoon

- All-purpose flour, three cups

- Brown sugar, three tablespoons

Instructions:

1. Place one cup of water and the next three ingredients in a bread machine pan in order. Set the setting for the dough. After 5 minutes of mixing, check the dough; add one to two tablespoons of water or flour if needed.

2. Turn the dough onto the gently floured surface when the cycle is finished. Split the dough into eight balls. Roll into a 20-inch rope; shape into pretzel type.

3. Preheat the stove to 425 °F. Bring two quarts of water with the baking soda to a boil in a wide saucepan. Drop the

pretzels, two at a time, into boiling water; cook for 10-15 seconds. With a slotted spoon, remove; drain onto paper towels.

4. Put pretzels on baking sheets that are oiled. Bake for 8-10 minutes, until golden brown. Spritz or spray gently with the remaining two tablespoons. Sprinkle salt on it.

Pumpkin Monkey Bread

Preparation Time: 45 minutes| **Servings:** 18 slices| **Difficulty: Medium**

Ingredients:

- Butter softened, two tablespoons

- Ground nutmeg, a quarter teaspoon

- All-purpose flour, 4 to four and a quarter cup

- Ground ginger, half teaspoon

- Ground cloves, a quarter teaspoon

- Active dry yeast, two teaspoons

- Sugar, a quarter cup

- Salt, one teaspoon

- Warm 2% milk (room temperature) one cup

- Canned pumpkin 3/4 cup

- The ground cinnamon, one teaspoon

Sauce:

- Canned pumpkin, a quarter cup

- The ground cinnamon, one teaspoon

- Butter cubed, one cup

- Packed brown sugar, one cup

- Dried cranberries, one cup

- Ground cloves, a quarter teaspoon

- Ground ginger, half teaspoon

- Ground nutmeg, a quarter teaspoon

Instructions:

1. Place the ingredients in the bread machine pan in the order recommended by the maker. Set the setting for the dough. After few minutes of mixing, check the dough; add one-two tablespoons of flour or water if necessary.

2. Meanwhile, mix the sauce ingredients in a broad saucepan; cook and stir until combined.

3. Turn the dough onto a gently floured surface until the dough step is finished. Break into 36 parts; mold into balls.

4. Arrange half of the 10-inch balls in an oiled pan with the fluted bowl; fill with half the sauce. Repeat, ensuring that the top layer is thoroughly covered with sauce.

5. Let rise until doubled, approximately 30 minutes in a warm spot.

6. Preheat the oven to 375°F. Bake for around 20-25 minutes, or till it turns golden brown. If the top browns very easily, cover loosely with tape.

7. Cool 10 minutes before serving. Serve it warm.

Blueberry Rolls

Preparation time:40 minutes|Servings:16 persons| Difficulty: Medium

Ingredients:

- One cup milk (room temperature)

- One large egg (room temperature)

- Two teaspoons of vanilla extract

- One tablespoon of active dry yeast

- 3/4 to one cup of blueberries (dried)

- Three and a half cups of all-purpose flour

- 1/3 cup of sugar

- One teaspoon of salt

- Four tablespoons of butter (softened; in small pieces)

- One tablespoon of water

- One large egg yolk

- One and a half cup of confectioners' sugar

- One tablespoon of butter (melted)

- One teaspoon of vanilla extract

- Two tablespoons of water (hot; or milk; plus, more for consistency)

- One teaspoon of cinnamon

Instructions:

1. Whisk the milk in a cup with the egg and vanilla extract.

2. The milk mixture, butter, flour, sugar, salt, and yeast are added to the bread maker pan in the order recommended by your machine maker.

3. Set the dough cycle, start the machine. At the beep, combine the blueberries and ground cinnamon.

4. Oil a round, 9-inch baking pan.

5. Turn and punch the dough out onto a floured surface. To prevent it from sticking to the surface and palms, knead a couple of times, adding a little more flour, if necessary.

6. Shape the dough into 16 identical balls and put them in the prepared round pan side-by-side. With a kitchen towel, cover the pan and let the rolls rise for 40 minutes in a draft-free spot.

7. Afterward, bake the rolls and serve.

Gruyère Apple Pie Cinnamon Buns with Vanilla Mocha Glaze

Preparation time: 2 hours 10 minutes|Servings: 12 persons| Difficulty: Hard

Ingredients:

- One teaspoon of lemon zest
- Three tablespoons of whipping the cream liquid
- One tablespoon of brewed French vanilla flavored coffee
- Two and a quarter cups of white flour
- Two tablespoons of sugar
- Half teaspoon of salt
- Half cup of grated Swiss Gruyere cheese
- Two teaspoons of bread making yeast
- Three tablespoons of whipped cream
- Three tablespoons of brown sugar
- A quarter cup of sliced almonds
- One teaspoon of cinnamon (ground)
- Two tablespoons of softened butter
- One and a half oz of cream
- Two tablespoons of water

- One egg large

- Three tablespoons of butter

- One cup of peeled green apples, cored and finely sliced (approximate two apples)

- A quarter cup of water

- One and a quarter cup of powdered sugar

- Two teaspoons of pure vanilla extract

Instructions:

1. Combine all the ingredients in the bread maker. Ensure the salt is added to one side of the bread pan and sugar to the other side. Dig a little well in the middle and apply the yeast in the end (do not let something touch it). Choose the dough cycle.

2. Transfer to a gently floured surface when the dough has finished (about 1 hour and 20 minutes). To make it easy to handle, knead enough (if necessary). If it is too elastic, let it rest for another 10 minutes.

3. Preheat the oven to 350°F. Spray with non-stick cooking spray on a 9×13 baking pan.

4. Meanwhile, mix the filling, slice the apples thinly and pour a quarter cup of water over them. Cook the apples in the

microwave for about three minutes until they are tender. Drain the water. Toss it with brown sugar, cinnamon, and almonds.

5. Roll the dough into a rectangle of 12×18. Spread softened butter on the dough. Cover with the mixture of apples and scatter uniformly over the butter. Evenly spread on top of the apple mixture the whipped cream. Roll up firmly like a jelly roll, beginning at the long end. Seal by a pinching seam. Cut into eight equal slices with a sharp knife and arrange in an oiled 9×13-inch baking sheet.

6. Cover the dough with a clean tea towel and let it rise until almost doubled in size in a warm, draft-free spot (30 minutes).

7. Bake the rolls for 25-30 minutes at 350° F or until baked.

8. Whipping cream and strong coffee are combined. Add the combination of vanilla and whipped cream to the sifted powdered sugar. Drizzle glaze over warm rolls once buns are finished. Serve cold or warm.

Chapter 2. Lunch Recipes

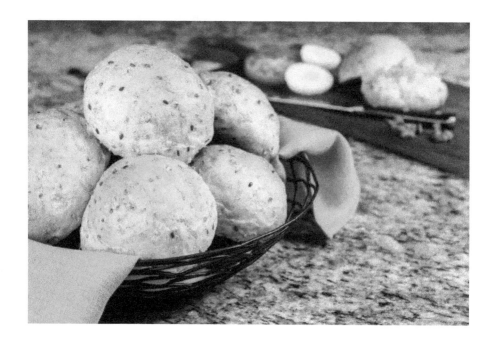

Flavorful Herb Bread

Preparation Time: 4 hours 15 minutes |Servings: 16 slices |Difficulty: Hard

Ingredients:

- Butter, two tablespoons

- Dried minced onion, a quarter cup

- Sugar, two tablespoons

- Warm whole milk (room temperature), one cup

- One large egg

- Salt, one and a half teaspoon

- Bread flour, three and a half cups

- Active dry yeast, two teaspoons

- Dried parsley flakes, two tablespoons

- Dried oregano, one teaspoon

Instructions:

1. Put all the ingredients in the bread machine's pan in the order recommended.

2. Pick the Basic Bread setting.

3. Bake according to the instructions, keep checking the dough every few minutes of mixing; use one to two tablespoons of water or flour if necessary.

Pepperoni Pizza

Preparation Time: 1 hour |Servings: 8 slices |Difficulty: Easy

Ingredients:

- Salt, one teaspoon

- All-purpose flour, three cups

- Active dry yeast, two and a half teaspoons

- One cup of cornmeal

- One tablespoon plus two tablespoons of water (room temperature)

- Grated Parmesan cheese, two tablespoons

- Olive oil, two tablespoons

- Italian seasoning, one and a half teaspoon

- Sugar, one teaspoon

Toppings:

- One package (8 ounces) sliced pepperoni

- Meatless spaghetti sauce, one cup

- Sugar, one to three teaspoons(optional)

- Two medium tomatoes, chopped

- Chopped onion, half cup

- Four cups of shredded part-skim mozzarella cheese

- Grated Parmesan cheese, half cup

- Italian seasoning, one and a half teaspoon

Instructions:

1. Place the first eight ingredients in the bread machine pan in the order suggested by the maker. Choose Dough Setup.

2. Turn the dough onto a gently floured surface when the cycle is finished. Roll into a 14-inch circle. Put it on an oiled cornmeal pizza plate. Move the dough to the prepared tray.

3. If needed, combine the spaghetti sauce and sugar; pour over the dough. Place the pepperoni, peppers, onion, cheese, and Italian seasoning on top.

4. Bake for 30-35 minutes at 400 °F or until the crust is finely browned. Before cutting, let it rest for 10 minutes.

Herbed Pesto Bread

Preparation Time: 2 hours 5 minutes |Servings: One loaf |Difficulty: Hard

Ingredients:

- Three cups of bread flour

- One and a half teaspoons of sugar

- One cup of water

- One teaspoon of salt

- A quarter cup of pesto sauce

- Two and a quarter teaspoons of bread machine yeast

- One teaspoon of lemon juice

Instructions:

1. Add all ingredients in the container of the bread machine in the suggested order by the manufacturer.

2. Select the basic cycle and size.

3. Press the start button and serve fresh.

Whole Wheat Pizza Dough with Honey

Preparation Time: 2 hours 10 minutes |Servings: 4 |Difficulty: Hard

Ingredients:

- Warm water, one cup

- Salt, one and a half teaspoon

- Whole wheat flour, one cup (120 grams or four and a quarter oz.)

- Honey, three-tablespoons

- Olive oil, two tablespoons

- Bread flour, two cups (240 grams)

- Bread machine or instant yeast, two teaspoons

Instructions:

1. In the order specified, bring all the ingredients into your bread machine. On the dough cycle, set the machine and click start.

2. Remove dough to a deep bowl (cover tightly) or pop dough into a large, zippered bag when the dough cycle ends and refrigerate overnight.

3. Remove the dough from the fridge for about an hour or two before you decide to bring your pizza together.

4. Divide in half and shape a smooth, rounded ball in half. At this point, in a well-oiled pizza pan, put each ball and cover it with plastic wrap.

5. Preheat the oven to 450° F until the dough has warmed up and it seems puffy.

6. To flatten the ball, use your hands and fingertips until it is the thickness you want. Use a 13-inch pie pan and lift it to the side.

7. In this order, arrange the pizza: first sauce, first cheese, then meat or other toppings.

8. Hop into the oven and adjust the temperature to 425°F. How long you bake the pizza based on how liberal you were with the toppings and the oven used. Watch after the first 10 minutes carefully.

Mini Maple Cinnamon Rolls

Preparation Time: 40 minutes |Servings: 26 |Difficulty: Easy

Ingredients:

- Whole milk, 2/3 cup

- One large egg

- Maple syrup, 1/3 cup

- Butter softened, 1/3 cup

- Salt, 3/4 teaspoon

- Bread flour, three cups

- Active dry yeast, one package (a quarter ounce)

Toppings:

- Packed brown sugar, half cup

- Bread flour, two tablespoons

- The ground cinnamon, four teaspoons

- Cold butter, six tablespoons

Maple Icing:

- Butter, three tablespoons

- Confectioners' sugar, one cup

- Maple syrup, three-tablespoons

- Whole milk, one to two teaspoons

Instructions:

1. Place the first seven ingredients in the bread machine pan in the order recommended by the maker. Pick Dough Setup.

2. Shift the dough on to a gently floured surface when the cycle is finished. Roll between two 12x7-inch, with rectangles. Combine brown sugar, flour, and cinnamon in a small bowl; cut into butter until the mixture is close to coarse crumbs. Over each rectangle, sprinkle percent. Starting with a long side, roll up jellyroll style, pinch seam to seal.

3. Split into 12 slices on each roll. In one oiled 13x9-inch, place cut side down in the pan for baking. Cover and let to rise until doubled, around 20 minutes, in a warm place.

4. Bake until golden brown, 20-25 minutes at 375°F. Cool for 5 minutes on a wire stand. Meanwhile, blend the sugar, butter, syrup, and milk in a small bowl to reach the perfect consistency. Pour over warm rolls.

Pumpkin Quick Bread

Preparation Time: 1 hour 20 minutes |Servings:16 |Difficulty: Medium

Ingredients:

- Three large eggs

- Pumpkin puree (canned or homemade), one and a half cups

- Granulated sugar, one cup

- Vegetable oil, 1/3 cup

- Ground nutmeg, a quarter teaspoon

- Ground ginger, a quarter teaspoon

- Baking powder, one and a half teaspoon

- Baking soda, half teaspoon

- A quarter teaspoon of salt

- The ground cinnamon, 3/4 teaspoon

- All-purpose flour, three cups

- Chopped walnuts or pecans (optional) half cup

Instructions:

1. Spray with baking spray on the bread machine pan.

2. Mix the sugar, vegetable oil, pumpkin puree, and eggs in a bowl until well mixed.

3. When mixed, whisk in baking powder, soda, cinnamon, seasoning, and flour.

4. Pour the prepared batter into the pan of the Bread Machine. Set it on the quick cycle of bread.

5. If desired, add in some chopped nuts when it beeps.

6. Loosen the loaf cautiously from the Bread Machine's pan and paddles and place it to cool out on a rack.

All Steak Orange Rolls

Preparation Time: 4 hours 30 minutes |Servings: 16 |Difficulty: Hard

Ingredients:

- One egg

- Six tablespoons of unsalted butter softened

- Three cups of all-purpose flour

- Heavy cream (warmed in the microwave for about 30 seconds) a quarter cup

- Frozen orange juice concentrate (thawed to room temperature) half cup

- Sugar, two tablespoons

- Salt, one teaspoon

- Two teaspoons of a bread machine or instant yeast

Filling:

- Unsalted butter softened, two tablespoons

- Sugar, half cup

- Orange zest (grated from two medium oranges) two tablespoons

Glaze:

- Heavy cream, a quarter cup

- Sugar, a quarter cup

- Orange juice concentrated, two tablespoons

- Unsalted butter, two tablespoons

- Salt, 1/8 teaspoon

Instructions:

1. In the order specified, add all the ingredients to the pan. Leave open the lid. Select the dough cycle and click start.

2. Observe the dough after 10 minutes or so. Add a tablespoon of water if the dough does not adhere to the pan's surface, then take it out when it is so dry. If the dough is too wet, apply a tablespoon of flour until the dough holds, then take it out. Keep adding flour or water until the dough is just right. Close the lid and allow for the completion of the dough cycle.

3. Check to see sure the dough twice the size after the dough cycle ends. If not, allow the dough to begin rising in the pan until the original volume is doubled.

4. Drop the dough on a floured surface from the bread machine pan. Roll into a shape measuring 12 x 17 inches or so.

5. Spread the softened butter over the rolled-out dough until it is completely coated in the dough. Sprinkle the combination of sugar and orange zest generously over the butter.

6. Start rolling the long-sided pastry. Roll as securely as possible. The large roll is cut into quarters. Split into five evenly sized rolls.

7. Place a buttered 9 x 13-inch pan inside, cover with a tea towel and enable to rise for around 45 minutes before baking in a warm place.

8. Preheat the oven to 325°F. Bake for 25-30 minutes or until the internal temperature exceeds 190°F.

9. Glaze prepared before baking rolls. Combine all the ingredients into a shallow saucepan, and under mixture heat over medium temperature becomes syrupy and covers the back of the spoon. Set to cool aside.

10. When they finish baking, spread the glaze over the hot rolls.

Braided Onion-Potato Loaf

Preparation Time: 40 minutes |Servings: 4 |Difficulty:
Easy

Ingredients:

- One large Yukon Gold potato peeled and cubed

- Honey, one tablespoon

- Grated Parmesan cheese, a quarter cup

- Chopped fresh parsley, a quarter cup

- Salt, one and a half teaspoon

- A quarter teaspoon of pepper

- One small onion, chopped

- One cup, warm 2% milk (room temperature)

- One large egg

- Butter, two tablespoons

- Bread flour, 4 cups

- Active dry yeast, one package (a quarter ounce)

Toppings:

- One large egg, lightly beaten.

- Additional grated Parmesan cheese

Instructions:

1. In a small saucepan, put the potato and onion and cover them with water. Just bring it to a simmer. Reduce heat; cover and cook until vegetables are tender or for 10-15 minutes. Drain; mash until smooth; set aside.

2. Place the milk, egg, parsley butter, sugar, cheese, mashed potato, salt, pepper, flour, and yeast in the bread machine pan in the order recommended by the maker. Pick the dough Setting.

3. Turn the dough onto a gently floured surface when the cycle is finished. Form each of them into an 18-inch rope—place ropes on an oiled baking sheet and braid, seal and tuck under by pinching ends.

4. Cover with a clean kitchen towel and rise until doubled, around 1 hour, in a warm spot. Uncover, top with a beaten egg brush. Bake for 25-35 minutes at 350°F or until golden brown. Remove from the pan on a rack to cool.

Calzone Rolls

Preparation Time:40 minutes |Servings:24 |Difficulty: Easy

Ingredients:

- Water (room temperature) one and 2/3 cups

- Salt, one and a quarter teaspoon

- All-purpose flour, four and a half cups

- Active dry yeast, two and a quarter teaspoon

- Nonfat dry milk powder, two tablespoons

- Sugar, two tablespoons

- Shortening, two tablespoons

- Chopped onion, half cup

- Diced pepperoni, half cup

- Shredded pizza cheese blend, one cup

- Chopped ripe olives. a quarter cup

- Sliced fresh mushrooms, half cup.

- Chopped green pepper, half cup

- Chopped sweet red pepper, half cup

- Olive oil, one tablespoon

- Pizza sauce, 1/3 cup

Instructions:

1. Place the first seven ingredients in the bread machine pan in the order recommended by the maker. Pick Dough Setting.

2. Sauté the onion, mushrooms, and peppers in oil until tender in a small skillet; then let it cool.

3. Turn the dough onto a gently floured surface when the bread machine cycle is completed; split by half. Let them rest for 5 minutes. Roll each section into a 16x10-inch rectangle piece; spread with sauce. Top with the combination of onion, pepperoni, pizza.

Onion French Bread Loaves

Preparation Time: 45 minutes |Servings:2 loaves |Difficulty: Medium

Ingredients:

- Water (room temperature) one cup

- Dried minced onion, half cup

- Active dry yeast, two and a quarter teaspoon

- Cornmeal, one tablespoon

- One large egg yolk, lightly beaten

- Sugar, one tablespoon

- Salt, two teaspoons

- Bread flour, three cups

Instructions:

1. Place the first six ingredients in the bread machine pan in order. Pick Dough Setting.

2. Turn the dough onto a gently floured surface when the cycle is finished. Cover and stop for 15 minutes to rest. Split the dough in two. Roll each section into a 15x10-inch piece for a square. Roll up the type of jellyroll, beginning with a long side, pinch to seal seams. The pinch ends up closing and tucking beneath.

3. Sprinkle an oiled baking sheet with the cornmeal. Place the loaves in a pan. Cover and enable to rise until doubled, around 30 minutes, in a warm place—egg yolk brush. Create two inches of 1/4-inch-deep cuts. It is separated from each loaf.

4. Bake for 20-25 minutes at 375°F or until golden brown. Remove from the pan to a rack.

5. Freeze option: Cover cooled loaves in heavy-duty foil tightly and freeze them. Place a foil-wrapped loaf on a baking sheet for use and reheat for 10-15 minutes in a 450°F oven. Remove the foil carefully; add to the crisp crust for a few minutes in the oven.

Garlic Herb Bubble Loaf

Preparation Time: 1 hour 20 minutes |Servings:18 |Difficulty: Medium

Ingredients:

- Butter softened, two tablespoons

- Sugar, three-tablespoons

- Salt, one and a half teaspoon

- Water, (room temperature) half cup

- Sour cream, half cup

- Bread flour, three cups

- Active dry yeast, two and a quarter teaspoon

Garlic Herb Butter:

- Four garlic cloves, minced

- Butter, (melted) a quarter cup

- Dried oregano, thyme, and rosemary crushed, each a quarter teaspoon

Instructions:

1. Place the first seven ingredients in the bread machine pan in the order recommended by the maker. Pick Dough Setting.

2. Turn the dough onto a gently floured surface when the cycle is finished. Cover and stop for 15 minutes to rest. Divide the dough into 36 separate parts. Form a ball into each piece.

3. Combine the butter, garlic, and spices in a small dish. Dip each ball in a mixture and put in an unoiled 9x5-inch pan. Cover and let rise until doubled, around 45 minutes, in a warm place.

4. Bake for 35-40 minutes at 375°F or until golden brown. Remove from the pan to a rack. Serve and enjoy.

Ciabatta Bread

Preparation time: 1 hour 5 minutes|Servings: 12 persons |Difficulty: Hard

Ingredients:

- One and a half cup of water

- Half teaspoon of salt

- One teaspoon of sugar

- One tablespoon of olive oil

- Three and a quarter cups of bread flour

- One and a half teaspoon of active dry yeast

Instructions:

1. Place all the ingredients in your bread machine's pan in the order required by your dough machine. Pick and launch the Dough Cycle.

2. To a countertop, apply a generous quantity of flour and put the dough on it. Then it is to be covered with plastic wrap and allow to rest for 20 minutes.

3. Divide the dough into two parts, with each forming a bread loaf shape. On a non-stick baking sheet, put the dough. Dust gently the flour on top.

4. Preheat the oven to 425° F. With a bottle of water, sprinkle the bread loaves with water. Bake for 25 to 30 minutes or until the bread is a little brown.

Wheat Berry Bread

Preparation time: 4 hours 30 minutes|Servings: 16 persons |Difficulty: Hard

Ingredients:

- One cup (240 grams) warm milk

- One and a half (6 grams) teaspoon of table salt

- One teaspoon (4 grams) of sugar

- Two tablespoons (28 grams) of unsalted butter, softened

- Half cup (160 grams) of whole-grain wheat berries

- Two and a half cups of bread flour, divided (300 grams)

- Two teaspoons (6 grams) of bread machine or instant yeast

Instructions:

1. Boil the wheat berries for 20 minutes in one cup of water. Let it cool (more rapidly if ice cubes are added) and drain. Alternatively, for 12 hours or overnight, soak the wheat berries in water. (The softened and drained wheat berries will last up to a week in the refrigerator.)

2. Add prepared wheat berries along with one cup of bread flour to a blender or food processor (120 grams). Process until you have finely chopped wheat berries.

3. Combine the milk or whey, salt, butter, sugar, remaining flour (180 grams), the mixture of ground-wheat-berries-and-flour, and the yeast.

4. Choose a cycle of dough and start. After 10 minutes, inspect the dough and ensure that the dough sticks to the pan's surface and then pulls away neatly. If it is too wet, apply one tablespoon more flour at a time. If it's too dry, use one tablespoon more water at a time.

5. Check to make sure the dough has doubled in size after the dough cycle ends. If not, keep it in the pan until it's finished.

6. Remove dough from pan to floured surface when doubled and divide into two equal parts. Pull dough from top to bottom until dough is smooth, form each portion into an oblong shape; then pinch closed on a baking sheet covered with a silicone mat. Otherwise, a parchment paper that has been coated with a touch of cornmeal put the seam side down.

7. Cover with a tea towel and leave it to rise until it nearly doubles. Preheat the oven to 425°F for about 20 minutes until the loaf is ready to bake.

8. Brush risen loaves with one egg white glaze whipped with one tablespoon sugar.

9. With a very sharp serrated knife or razor blade, make two-three diagonal slashes in each loaf, careful not to deflate the dough.

10. Bake for 20-25 minutes in a preheated oven, or until the interior temperature touches 190° F, or until the bottom is brown and sounds hollow.

11. Allow the loaves to cool for an hour on the rack before slicing.

Chapter 3. Dinner Recipes

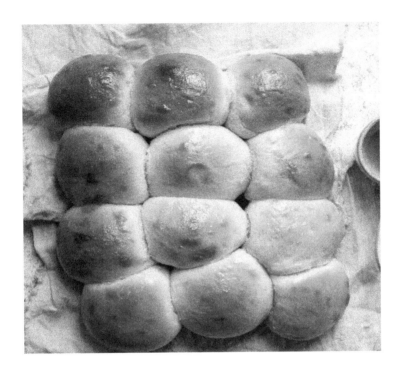

Hamburger Buns

Preparation Time: 25 minutes |Servings: 8 |Difficulty: Easy

Ingredients:

- Water, one and 1/3 cups

- Salt, two teaspoons

- Nonfat milk powder, two tablespoons

- All-purpose flour, four cups (a little more for kneading)

- Shortening, two tablespoons

- Sugar, two and a half plus three tablespoons

- Active dry yeast, two and a half teaspoons

- Cornmeal

- Sesame seeds, two tablespoons

Instructions:

1. Gather all the ingredients.

2. Add some water and nonfat milk powder to the bread machine, followed by the flour. Keep the cycle to "dough" and add shortening and the salt, yeast, and sugar.

3. The dough cycle is done, put the dough out onto a floured board and punch it down. Knead it 4 or 5 times; you can add

a little more flour as you knead it necessary to keep the dough from sticking to the board or your fingers.

4. Cover up the dough with a clean dishcloth and let it rest for about half an hour.

5. Slightly butter a large baking sheet, sprinkle on some cornmeal.

6. Pat the dough in a circle and cut it into eight wedges. Make each wedge into a ball, then flatten each one in a smooth, fairly even circle, slightly a little bigger than a burger.

7. Arrange those dough pieces onto the baking sheet about two inches apart and let it rest for 20 minutes.

8. Preheat the oven at 375° F.

9. Slightly brush the buns with some egg wash and sprinkle with sesame seeds or poppy seeds.

10. Bake the buns for 20 minutes till the buns are completely ready.

11. Let it cool for some time before serving.

Jewish Challah

Preparation Time: 45 minutes |Servings: 16 |Difficulty: Medium

Ingredients:

- Salt, one and a half teaspoon

- Honey, half cup

- Oil (vegetable) two and a half tablespoon

- Flour (bread) four and a 2/3 cups

- One large egg (beaten)

- One large egg yolk (beaten)

- Water (lukewarm) one cup

- Large egg (beaten for egg wash) one

- Sesame/poppy seeds

- Yeast (instant or bread machine) one and a quarter teaspoon

Instructions:

1. Add salt, egg yolk, water, egg, honey, and put oil on the bread pan. Add yeast and spoon flour on top of the liquid.

2. Press Start and Select the Sweet or Basic/White cycle and the Light Crust setting.

3. Pause, and at the start of the final rise, remove dough from the bread pan, transfer to a lightly floured surface & punch it down.

4. Divide dough into thirds. Into a 10-inches long rope, roll each third. On the floured surface parallel to each other, lay the three strings out, so very close they are but not touching each other. Braid together the ropes snugly. Tuck ends under for forming a long loaf.

5. With beaten egg, brush the braid & sprinkle with poppy seeds, pressing the seeds into the dough.

6. From the bread pan, remove kneading paddle(s). Put braid in the pan and click start to continue the cycle.

7. Place the bread on a wire rack when it is ready to cool completely before slicing.

Meat Pizza Dough

Preparation Time: 45 minutes |Servings: 16 |Difficulty: Easy

Ingredients:

- Salt, one and a half teaspoon

- Active dry yeast, one and a half teaspoon

- Water, one and a half cups

- Bread flour, three and 3/4 cups

- Olive oil/ Vegetable oil, one and a half tablespoon

- Granulated sugar, one tablespoon plus one teaspoon

Instructions:

1. Gather all the ingredients.

2. In the order recommended, add the ingredients to the bread machine. Choose the dough cycle.

3. Take the dough out and fit into pizza pans and roll it out to form an an-inch-thick edge.

4. Preheat oven to 400° F.

5. With olive oil or vegetable oil, lightly brush the dough, and then let the crust rise for about 10 to 15 minutes. Spread toppings of choice and with the tomato sauce.

6. About 25 minutes, bake pizza in the oven until the crust is ready and cheese has melted properly.

7. Slice the pizza and enjoy.

Garlic Pizza Dough

Preparation Time: 50 minutes |Servings: 16 |Difficulty: Easy

Ingredients:

- One and a half cups of water

- Three minced garlic cloves

- One and a half tablespoons of vegetable oil (or olive oil)

- Three and 3/4 cups of bread flour

- Half cup of grated cheese of your choice

- One tablespoon plus one teaspoon sugar (granulated)

- One and a half teaspoons of salt

- One and a half teaspoons of active dry yeast

Instructions:

1. In the order prescribed by the manufacturer, add ingredients to your bread machine. Choose the duration of the dough.

2. To fit into pizza pans, remove the dough and stretch it out, creating a one-inch-thick lip.

3. Preheat the oven to 400° F

4. Brush the crust with a small amount of olive oil or vegetable oil, and let it rise for 10-15 minutes. Spread with tomato sauce or your choice of toppings.

5. Bake for 20 to 25 minutes in the oven or until the crust is browned and the cheese is melted and sparkling. Serve and enjoy.

Kalamata Olive Bread

Preparation Time: 2 hours 10 minutes |Servings: 10 |Difficulty: Medium

Ingredients:

- Brine from olives 1/3 to half cup

- Warm water, one cup

- Olive oil, two tablespoons

- Bread flour, three cups

- Wheat flour, one and 2/3 cups

- Salt, one and a half teaspoon

- Sugar, two tablespoons

- Basil, (dried leaf) one and a half teaspoon

- Active dry yeast, two teaspoons

- Olives (finely chopped kalamata, about two dozen pitted olives) half to 2/3 cup

Instructions:

1. On a two-cup scale, place the olive brine; put warm water to create the amount of one and a half cups.

2. According to your maker's desired order, place the ingredients in the bread machine, except for the olives.

3. Pick your bread machine's simple or wheat mode.

4. At the beep of your bread machine, add olives and add the mix-in ingredients.

5. Slice it and enjoy it with olive oil or with butter when your loaf is done baking.

Whole Wheat Crescent Dinner Rolls

**Preparation Time: 1 hour 30 minutes |Servings: 16
|Difficulty: Medium**

Ingredients:

- A quarter cup of slivered blanched almonds

- Two cups of whole wheat flour

- One cup of water

- Two large eggs

- Four tablespoons, unsalted butter, cut into pieces

- Half cup of sour cream

- Two and a quarter cups of bread flour

- Two tablespoons of light brown sugar

- One tablespoon of gluten

- Two teaspoons of salt

- Two and 3/4 teaspoons of bread machine yeast

Instructions:

1. Place them in a dry skillet with the almonds. Lightly toast
   over medium heat, stirring continuously, for two minutes or
   so. Combine the almonds in a food processor with two
   teaspoons of whole wheat flour. Grind it for a decent dinner.

2. As per the manufacturer's instructions, put all ingredients, including the almond meal, in the pan.

3. Set the settings of the Dough Cycle Program; Click Start.

4. Top the parchment paper with two baking sheets. Turn the dough out directly on a lightly floured work surface as the machine beeps at the end of the cycle; split it into two separate parts. Roll each section into a 10-inch round with a rolling pin. Slice each round into eight pie-shaped wedges using a pastry wheel. At the base of the triangle, roll up each wedge from the broad edge and position the crescents one-inch apart on the baking sheet, point-side down. Cover gently with plastic wrap and grow until almost doubled in bulk, about 30 minutes, at room temperature.

5. Preheat the oven to 375°F twenty minutes before baking.

6. Bake the rolls for 15 to 18 minutes, one pan at a time, or until lightly browned. Let it partly cool on a shelf. Eat the rolls warmly.

Rose Rolls with Rose Buttercream

Preparation Time: 1 hour 30 minutes |Servings: 16 |Difficulty: Medium

Ingredients:

For the dough:

- 3/4 cup of milk

- Half cup of water

- One large egg

- Half cup of (one stick) unsalted butter, cut into pieces

- Four cups of unbleached all-purpose flour

- Half cup of sugars

- Two teaspoons of salt

- One tablespoon of bread machine yeast

For the filling:

- Two and ¾ cup of cherry pie filling

For the rose buttercream:

- One cup of sifted confectioners' sugar

- Pinch of salt

- Two tablespoons of warm milk

- Half teaspoon of vanilla extract or one and a quarter teaspoons vanilla powder added to the sugar

- Half teaspoon of rose water, optional

- One and a half tablespoons of unsalted butter, room temperature

Instructions:

1. In order to make the dough, according to the manufacturer's directions, put all the dough ingredients in the bowl.

2. Select the Dough Cycle Program; Click Start. The ball of dough would be soft. Click Pause and unplug the machine if the machine beeps at the end of the loop. Turn out the dough and mold it into a thick square that will fit into a 4-quart plastic bucket that is oiled. Cover with plastic tape, and refrigerate overnight or for 2 hours.

3. Line two parchment paper baking sheets. To deflate it, softly press the dough and place it on a lightly floured work surface. Roll out the dough into a 12-by-16-by-14-inch rectangle. Break the dough lengthwise with a sharp knife or pastry wheel into 16 one-inch-wide strips. Twist one in the opposite direction from the other at the same time by placing your hands on either end of a strip. Wrap the whole strip to create a coiled pinwheel at one end. Tuck beneath the tail. For the other strips of dough, repeat.

4. Place the pinwheels on the baking sheets at least two inches apart (8 per pan). Do not crowd. Cover with plastic wrap and set aside to rise at room temperature until doubled in bulk, One to one and a half hours.

5. Preheat the oven to 400°F.

6. Using your fingertips, gently press to the bottom of each coil's center to form an indentation for the filling. Place about two tablespoons of the pie filling into the center. Be careful not to use too much filling, or it will bubble over during baking. You want filling surrounded by dough.

7. Place a second baking sheet of the same dimensions under one of the pans holding pastries to double pan and prevent the bottoms from burning. Bake for 13 to 16 minutes. Remove the pan from the oven and place it on a wire rack. Double pan and place the second batch of rolls in the oven.

8. As the second batch bakes, frost the first batch. Make the buttercream frosting by mixing all the frosting ingredients together in a small bowl; beat until smooth and thick, yet pourable. Glaze the pastries while still warm and on the baking sheet, drizzling the glaze back and forth with the end of a spoon, a pastry bag fitted with a small plain tip, or the tips of your fingers. Move the pastries from the baking pan to a wire rack to cool. The frosting will set as it cools. When the second batch of rolls is finished, frost the same way. Let the pastries cool on the racks for 15 minutes before eating.

Sun-Dried Tomato and Olive Loaf

Preparation Time: 50 minutes |Servings: 16 |Difficulty: Easy

Ingredients:

- Warm tomato juice (room temperature) one cup

- Olive oil, two tablespoons

- Salt, half teaspoon

- Brown sugar, two teaspoons

- Minced fresh rosemary or one teaspoon dried rosemary, crushed, one tablespoon

- Bread flour, two and a 3/4 cups

- Quick-rise yeast, one package (a quarter ounce)

- Chopped oil-packed sun-dried tomatoes, well-drained, half cup

- Chopped pitted Greek olives, well-drained, half cup

Instructions:

1. Add tomato juice, one tablespoon oil, salt, flour, brown sugar, rosemary, and yeast into a bread machine in the order indicated by the maker. Pick the setting for the dough. After 5 minutes of mixing, check the dough; add one-two tablespoons of water or flour if required. Put the tomatoes

and olives before kneading it (the system can audibly signal this).

2. Gently, turn the dough on a floured surface when the cycle is finished. Roll it into a 15x10-inch oval shape. Roll up into a jelly-roll style, starting from a long side. Poke the seam to seal and tuck the ends. Put it on a baking sheet upside side down.   Cover the rolls with a towel; leave it to rise twice its size, about 45 minutes, in a warm spot—Preheat the oven to 400° F.

3. Brush the bread with oil. Create five wide slashes through the top of the bread with a knife. Bake for around 20-25 minutes, till it turns golden brown. To cool, transfer it from the pan to a wire rack.

Hawaiian Dinner Rolls

Preparation Time: 1 hour 10 minutes |Servings: 15 rolls |Difficulty: Medium

Ingredients:

- Water (room temperature) a quarter cup

- Sugar, one tablespoon

- Salt, one and a half teaspoon

- Crushed pineapple, undrained one can (8 ounces)

- Bread flour, three and a quarter cup

- Warm pineapple juice (room temperature) a quarter cup

- Sweetened shredded coconut, 3/4 cup

- One large egg

- Butter, cubed, a quarter cup

- Active dry yeast, two and a quarter teaspoon

- Nonfat dry milk powder, a quarter cup

Instructions:

1. Place the first ten ingredients in the bread machine pan in the order recommended by the maker. Pick Dough Setup. Add coconut just before final kneading (your system can audibly signal this).

---

2. Turn the dough onto a gently floured surface when the cycle is finished, cover for 10 minutes to rest. Break into 15 parts; roll each one into a ball. Place them in a 13x9-inch oiled pan for baking.

3. Cover and let it rise for 45 minutes or until doubled in a warm spot. Bake for 15-20 minutes at 375°F or till it turns golden brown.

Meat Pizza Dough

Preparation   Time:2   hours |Servings:6
|Difficulty: Hard

Ingredients:

- Springwater, one cup, and one tablespoon

- Salt, one teaspoon

- Honey, one tablespoon

- Granulated sugar, one teaspoon

- Bread flour, three cups (360 gr)

- Olive oil, two tablespoons

- Fast-rising or bread machine yeast, two and a quarter teaspoon

Instructions:

1. In the order specified, put the ingredients in the bread machine. Pick the dough cycle.

2. After 5 minutes, check the dough. It's expected to gather into a ball that is sticking to the pan's side, then pulls free. Add a tablespoon of flour if it does not come away despite sticking.

3. Preheat the oven to 500° F.

4. Remove the dough from the pan to a floured surface until the dough cycle finishes and pizza dough is twice the size. Break

into two bits and form into a ball every half. Cover for 10-15 minutes to rise.

5. Spray two heavy pizza pans or a baking sheet with oil (use two 13-inch circular pans). Place and cajole pizza with your hands to the perfect thinness. The usage of a rolling pin helps to compress the dough. If the dough is stretch-resistant, let it rest and chill for a couple of minutes, then get back to it.

6. Second, layer sauce (do not overdo it), yogurt, and meat or vegetables afterward. Excess toppings will make it too long for your pizza to bake and result in a soggy base.

7. In a preheated oven, roast it. Once you put the pizza in, turn the temperature up to 450° F. Bake for 10-15 minutes or until the crust on the edges is white and the cheese on top of the pizza turns golden brown in places.

8. Let cool for two-three minutes, enjoy.

Quick and Soft Dinner Rolls

Preparation Time: 55 minutes |Servings: two dozens |Difficulty: Medium

Ingredients:

- Water, (room temperature) one cup

- Sugar, a quarter cup

- One large egg

- Salt, one and a quarter teaspoon

- Butter, cubed, a quarter cup

- Nonfat dry milk powder, three-tablespoons

- Bread flour, three and a quarter cup

- Quick-rise yeast one package (a quarter ounce)

- Egg wash- one large egg

Instructions:

1. Place the first eight ingredients in the bread machine pan in the order recommended. Pick the setting for the dough. After 5 minutes of mixing, check the dough; add one-two tablespoons of water or flour if required.

2. Gently, turn the dough on a floured surface when the cycle is finished. Divide into 24 balls and shape them. Roll into an 8-inch rope; tie into a loose knot.

3. Put one and a half aside on oiled baking sheets. Cover with a towel; let it rise twice in a warm place, about 30 minutes.

4. Preheat the oven to 400 ° F.

5. Whisk the egg and water in a small bowl for egg wash; brush over the rolls—Bake for eight to nine minutes. Remove from pans to racks of wire; serve warm.

Sour Cream Chia Bread

Preparation Time: 1 hour 10 minutes |Servings: 16 |Difficulty: Medium

Ingredients:

- Water, (room temperature) a quarter cup

- Whole milk, (room temperature)2/3 cup

- Sour cream, a quarter cup

- Butter, two tablespoons

- Minced chives, a quarter cup

- Salt, one and a half teaspoon

- Sugar, one and a half teaspoon

- Bread flour, three cups

- Baking soda, 1/8 teaspoon

- Active dry yeast, two and a quarter teaspoon

Instructions:

1. Place all ingredients in the order proposed by the manufacturer in the bread machine tray.

2. Pick the simple setting for the bread. If available, choose the crust color and loaf size.

3. Bake as directed by the bread machine.

Cajun Bread

Preparation Time: 1 hour 30 minutes |Servings: 12|Difficulty: Medium

Ingredients:

- Sugar, one tablespoon

- Water, half cup

- Salt, half teaspoon (use about 3/4 teaspoon if your Cajun seasoning is salt-free)

- Onion, (chopped) a quarter cup

- Garlic, (chopped finely) two teaspoons

- Butter, (soft) two teaspoons

- Green bell pepper, (chopped) a quarter cup

- Bread flour, two cups

- Cajun (or creole) seasoning, one teaspoon

- Active dry yeast, one teaspoon

Instructions:

1. Similar to the manufacturer's instructions for inserting ingredients, weigh all ingredients in the machine.

2. Choose the base/white bread cycle. Use the hue of a light or dark crust. (Do not use loops for delays.)

3. Take the bread out and cool on the rack with wire.

Instructions on Sandwich Roll:

1. Place the components in the bread machine and select the configuration for the dough.

2. Take out the dough from the machine, cut it into roughly 10 to 12 pieces, and mold it into rolls.

3. Put them on a wide baking sheet that is loosely oiled or lined with parchment paper.

4. Cover with a moist towel and allow the rolls to grow for 35 to 45 minutes or until they have doubled.

5. Whisk an egg white with one tablespoon of water just before baking, then brush over each roll.

6. Sprinkle, with sesame seeds, if needed.

7. Bake for around 15 minutes in a preheated 350° F oven, or until golden brown.

Chapter 4. Dessert Recipes

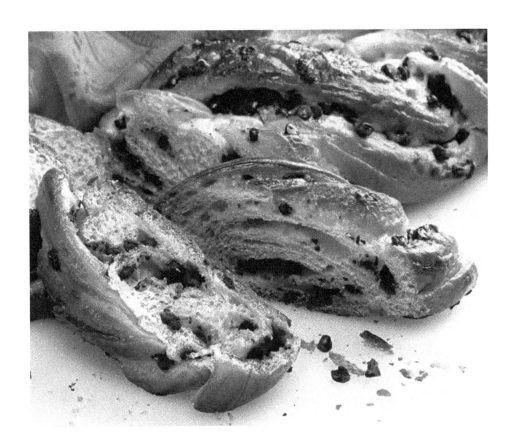

Sweet Banana Bread with Yeast

Preparation Time: 3 hours 30 minutes |Servings: 6 |Difficulty: Hard

Ingredients:

- One large egg

- Warm milk or yogurt, 1/3 cup

- Honey, one tablespoon

- Salt, half teaspoon

- Butter, two tablespoons

- Ripe banana, mashed (approximately half cup or 5 ounces)

- Wheat flour, one cup (120 g)

- Bread flour (can substitute all-purpose unbleached) one and ¾ cup (210g)

- Bread-machine or instant yeast, two teaspoons (8g)

- Toasted pecans or almonds, half c. (65 g)

- Raisins, 1/3 c. (50 g)

- Chopped dates, a quarter c. (45g)

Topping:

- Ground cardamom, half teaspoon

- One tablespoon of milk

- One tablespoon of sugar

Instructions:

1. In the order specified, mix all of the dough ingredients into a bread-machine pan (except the raisins, nuts, and dates). Set on the dough period. Add nuts and dried fruit.

2. When the dough has expanded to twice its size at the end of the period, extract the pan's dough. Keep the dough in the machine till it starts to rise. Remove to a surface that is gently floured and shape into a ball. Give 10 minutes for the dough ball to rest.

3. Split it into three separate parts. Create three cylinders 12 inches long each. Braid, tucking the ends underneath.

4. Move to a parchment paper-covered cookie sheet or a silicone baking pad. Lined with a tea towel, let rise for about 45 minutes. (If you are frightened by the principle of braiding, cut the dough into three balls and put it in a loaf pan side by side.)

5. Lightly wipe milk over the lifted bread. Combine the cardamom sugar and scatter it on top of the braid.

6. Bake for 30-35 minutes or until cooked at 375°F.

7. Note: Until the loaf in the middle is baked, cover the loaf with foil to prevent the top crust from over-browning. If you have a digital quick-read thermometer, which is suggested to

make a ton of bread, the temperature should be around 190 °
F.

Cranberry Sauce Rolls

Preparation Time: 3 hours 15 minutes |Servings: 16 | Difficulty: Hard

Ingredients:

- One cup of jellied cranberry sauce, at room temperature

- A quarter cup of lukewarm whole milk or half and half

- One egg

- One cup of dried cranberries

- One teaspoon of salt

- A quarter cup of butter softened

- Two medium lemons

- Three cups of all-purpose unbleached flour

- Two teaspoons of bread machine yeast

Instructions:

1. In the order specified, add all the ingredients to the machine.

2. Pick the duration of the dough and press the start button.

3. Put cranberries into the dough as the machine beeps to signal the right moment for additions.

4. Remove the dough and put it on a floured surface when the dough cycle is over.

5. Divide the dough into two identical parts. Divide each of these dough balls into eight pieces of the same size and form them into balls.

6. Place balls into two 8-inch cake cups.

7. Cover the rolls with tea towels, let them grow for around 45 minutes or until they are almost doubled.

8. Preheat the oven to 350°C.

9. Bake for around 14-16 minutes, or until golden brown.

10. Let the rolls stay in the pan for around 5-8 minutes after extracting the oven rolls. To cool, transfer on a wire rack.

Bread Bear Claws

Preparation Time: 3 hours |Servings:8 |Difficulty: Hard

Ingredients:

- Warm water, a quarter cup

- Sour cream, a quarter cup

- Sugar, a quarter cup

- Salt, half teaspoon

- One egg

- Butter, (softened) a quarter cup

- All-purpose, unbleached flour, two and a quarter cup and one tablespoon (280 g)

- Bread machine yeast, two teaspoons

Filling:

- Sugar, a quarter cup

- Cinnamon, one teaspoon

- Softened butter, two tablespoons

Frosting:

- Butter, two teaspoons

- Cream cheese, two teaspoons

- Coffee or milk, one and a half tablespoon

- Powdered sugar, one cup

- Toasted sliced almonds, a quarter cup

Instructions:

1. In the order mentioned, add the ingredients to a machine pan. Set the dough cycle. Remove the dough from the pan until done.

2. On a lightly floured board, roll the dough in a rectangle measuring 6 x 24 inches.

3. On the square pan, scatter the softened butter. Sprinkle generously around the buttered region with the cinnamon and sugar mixture.

4. Start rolling and roll tightly as necessary. Slightly flatten the log with your hands and break the log into ten parts.

5. Create two cuts through each slice of a pizza cutter, slicing half-inch of all the other side.

6. To make it lie much flatter, curl each slice slightly. Place it on an oiled baking sheet or one filled with a silicone mat or parchment paper.

7. Cover and watch it rise before it almost doubles. (45 minutes to 1 hour)

8. Bake the rolls until golden brown for 15-20 minutes at 375° F.

Frosting:

1. Soften the cream cheese and butter or make them reach room temperature. Mix the cream cheese, butter, and milk, or coffee and beat until completely smooth.

2. To drizzle frosting on the rolls, use a spoon. Or pour the frosting into a tiny, zippered plastic container. Slice off a tiny corner on the bag and drizzle the frosting back over the rolls using the closed pocket.

3. Immediately scatter toasted almonds on frosted rolls until the frosting dries.

4. Take the frosted roll and turn it upside down, pouring the icing onto an almond tray. This means that the icing would adhere to the almonds.

Cinnamon Roll using the Tangzhong

Preparation Time: 2 hours 40 minutes |Servings: 16 | Difficulty: Hard

Ingredients:

Dough:

- Milk divided, one cup

- One tablespoon of heavy cream or one egg yolk

- Sugar, one tablespoon

- Unbleached flour divided into three cups

- Four tablespoons of softened butter and four tablespoons for the filling

- One egg

- Salt, a quarter teaspoon

- Instant yeast, one teaspoon

Filling:

- Brown sugar, 3/4 cup

- Cinnamon, one teaspoon

- Pinch of ground cloves

- Chopped, toasted pecans (optional) half cup

Icing:

- Powdered sugar, two cups

- Softened cream cheese, one ounce

- Coffee (leftover or instant is good enough) or milk, two tablespoons

Instructions:

1. Measure one cup of milk.

2. Measure out a tiny bowl of three cups of unbleached flour.

3. Measure and split four teaspoons of butter into small pieces. Set it aside to reach room temperature.

4. Create a paste mixture in a medium-sized microwave-safe jar by whisking half the milk (half cup) and three tablespoons of flour together. Cook for one minute on high, whisking after 30 seconds, then after 15 seconds, again. Like pudding, the paste should be dense.

5. Apply the paste mixture along with the remaining half cup of milk to the bread-machine pan.

6. In the bread machine pan, add the milk, salt, sugar, cream or softened butter, egg yolk, yeast, and remaining pre-measured flour and pick the dough cycle. Click "Start."

7. Remove from the pan, softly punch down, and split the dough into half if it has risen to twice its original size. Roll

each half into a rectangle of around 13 x 10 inches on a generously floured board.

8. With two tablespoons of softened butter or heavy cream, spread each rectangle.

Filling:

1. Combine the brown sugar, cinnamon, and cloves.

2. Spread half of the mixture over the rectangle and half on the next rectangle. Sprinkle quarter pecans cover the cinnamon layer, sliced, toasted.

3. Roll the long way up the dough. Cut into eight identical slices. Set the cut side down into an 8-inch oiled pan or glass dish.

4. In a soft, moist spot, cover and let rise until nearly double.

5. Around 15 minutes until the rolls are ready to bake, set the oven to 375° F. Preheat it.

6. Bake the rolls for 20 minutes or until they are golden brown.

Frosting:

1. Ice with a blend of two cups of powdered sugar, one ounce of cream cheese, and two tablespoons of coffee. Depending on how dense the icing is, you can need more or less milk.

Basic Cinnamon Rolls

Preparation Time: 2 hours 15 minutes |Servings :12 |Difficulty: Hard

Ingredients:

For the Dough:

- Bread flour, three and a 1/3 cups

- Milk, one cup

- Butter (half stick of margarine) a quarter cup

- One large egg

- Sugar, three-tablespoons

- Active dry yeast, two teaspoons

- Salt, half teaspoon

For the Filling:

- Butter (melted), a quarter cup

- Nuts (chopped and lightly toasted), 1/3 cup

- Sugar, a quarter cup

- Cinnamon, two teaspoons

- Nutmeg, half teaspoon

For the Icing:

- Powdered sugar, one cup

- Milk, one to two tablespoons

- Vanilla extract, half teaspoon

Instructions:

1. Collect ingredients.

2. As suggested by the maker, add wheat, milk, butter, egg, sugar, yeast, and salt to your bread machine for the dough. Set the dough cycle and let the machine do its work.

3. Place the dough on a floured surface until the process is finished. For around a minute, knead the dough, rest it another 15 minutes.

Filling:

1. Roll out the dough, about 15 by 10 centimeters, into a rectangle.

2. Over the dough, brush a quarter cup of melted butter within one inch of the sides.

3. In a cup, add together the diced almonds, butter, cinnamon, and nutmeg. Sprinkle generously over the dough with the mixture.

4. Roll the dough up firmly, beginning on the long side. To seal and mold into a 12-inch-long, uniformly rounded roll, push the sides.

5. Cut the whole roll into one-inch bits using a knife or an 8-inch-long strip of uncoated dental floss.

Rising and Baking:

1. Grease a baking sheet that is 13 x 9 inches.

2. Place cut side down rolls in the bowl. Cover and let grow until they double in size in a warm, draft-free spot. It's going to take around 30 to 45 minutes.

3. Preheat the oven to 375° F.

4. For around 20 to 25 minutes or until golden brown, bake the rolls.

Frost and the Coating:

1. Collect all the ingredients.

2. In a bowl, combine the sugar syrup, milk, and vanilla. Blend the mixture until smooth. Add more powdered sugar or milk, whether it is too thin or too dense before the perfect consistency is met.

3. Cool the rolls for 10 to 15 minutes in the bowl, then drizzle them with the powdered icing sugar.

Blueberry Rolls

Preparation Time: 1 hour 50 minutes |Servings: 16 |Difficulty: Medium

Ingredients:

- One large egg (at room temperature)

- Vanilla extract, two teaspoons

- Milk, (room temperature) one cup

- All-purpose flour, three and a half cups

- Butter, (softened; in small pieces) four tablespoons

- Sugar, 1/3 cup

- Salt, one teaspoon

- Active dry yeast, one tablespoon

- Blueberries, (dried) 3/4 to one cup

- Cinnamon, one teaspoon

- Water, one tablespoon

- One large egg yolk

For the Vanilla Icing:

- One and a half cups of confectioners' sugar

- One tablespoon of butter (melted)

- One teaspoon of vanilla extract

- Two tablespoons of hot water or milk; plus, more for consistency

Instructions:

1. Whisk the milk with the egg and vanilla extract in a mug.

2. Add the milk mixture, sugar, flour, butter salt, and yeast to the bread machine pan in the order recommended by the machine's maker.

3. Set the dough cycle, start the machine. Use a beep to insert the blueberries and ground cinnamon.

4. Grease a rectangular 9-inch baking sheet.

5. On a floured board, turn out the dough and punch it flat. To prevent it from sticking to the surface and palms, knead a couple of times, adding a little more flour, if appropriate.

6. In the prepared circular pan, shape the dough into 16 standardized balls and put them side-by-side. Cover the pan with a kitchen towel and allow the rolls to rise for 40 minutes in a draft-free location.

7. Preheat oven to 350° F.

8. Whisk the water and egg yolk into a shallow bowl. Brush over the tops of the rolls with the mixture.

9. The rolls are golden brown for 20 to 25 minutes, or before the tops are golden brown.

10. Remove the rolls to a rack and allow them to cool for 5 to 10 minutes while the icing is being prepared.

11. Combine the pastries' sugar in a cup with the melted butter and one teaspoon of vanilla extract. Apply two tablespoons of hot water or milk, or sufficiently to achieve a decent quality of drizzling.

12. From the tray, move the rolls to a rack. Put a sheet under the rack with foil or wax paper.

13. Drizzle over the soft rolls with the icing.

Glazed Yeast Doughnuts

Preparation Time: 10 hours 25 minutes |Servings: 24 slices |Difficulty: Hard

Ingredients:

- Evaporated milk, half cup

- One egg (beaten)

- Water, half cup

- Salt, one teaspoon

- Active dry yeast, two teaspoons

- Oil for deep-frying

- Butter, two tablespoons

- Sugar, 1/3 cup

- All-purpose flour, three cups

For the Chocolate Glaze:

- Two tablespoons of butter

- Two tablespoons of cocoa

- Three tablespoons of hot water

- One and a half cups of powdered sugar

- Half teaspoon of vanilla extract

Instructions:

1. Using the bread machine to combine components. Cover the pan with plastic wrap after the kneading period, then move it to the refrigerator. (Or, into a loosely oiled bowl,)

2. Overnight, refrigerate.

3. Remove the dough to a lightly floured surface and roll to a thickness of around half -inch.

4. Break the knots or cruller forms out into doughnut shapes or type strips. Cover and let grow for approximately 1 hour.

5. Fry at 360°F in oil until light and brown. Glaze with the chocolate coloring that accompanies or use your preferred coating.

Glaze with Chocolate or Vanilla:

1. Melt butter over low heat in a small saucepan; add cocoa and water.

2. Stir continually until the mixture is dense.

3. Remove from heat; combine powdered sugar and vanilla gradually; beat until smooth with a whisk.

4. Add half a teaspoon of extra hot water at a time before the quality is drizzling.

5. To glaze the vanilla, omit the cocoa and apply one and a half teaspoon of vanilla.

Chocolate Bread

Preparation Time: 3 hours 15 minutes |Servings: 8 |Difficulty: Hard

Instructions:

- Whole milk, half cup

- Sugar, 1/3 cup

- Unsweetened dark cocoa powder, three tablespoons

- Salt, one teaspoon

- Eggs, two

- Butter (half stick), softened a quarter cup

- Greek yogurt (or sour cream) a quarter cup

- Vanilla extract, one teaspoon

- Three cups of bread flour (360 grams)

- Bread machine or instant yeast, two teaspoons

Filling:

- Butter, (very soft) a quarter cup

- Brown sugar, half cup

- Cinnamon, one teaspoon

- Pecans, (toasted) half cup

Icing:

- Unsweetened chocolate, one and a half ounces

- Vanilla extract, one teaspoon

- Milk, two tablespoons

- Butter, one tablespoon

- Powdered sugar (sifted if it has lumps) one and a half cup

Instructions:

1. In the order specified, put some dough ingredients on the pan. Set it On the Dough loop, configure your machine, and press start.

2. Open the lid after 10-15 minutes and determine the dough's consistency. If the dough becomes too sticky, apply one tablespoon of flour at a time to shape a pliable ball. If it is so dry and the side is pounded, use one tablespoon of milk at a time. The dough can adhere to the side and then be cleanly taken away.

3. Lift the dough from the pan onto a well-floured board when the dough cycle is full, and the dough has risen to twice its original size.

4. Mold the dough into just a ball. Cut in two. Roll every half into a square measuring 11 x 11-inch.

5. Over the end, scatter half (two tablespoons) of butter. Sprinkle half the combination of brown sugar and cinnamon equally over all the butter, then half the diced pecans.

6. Roll the dough beginning from one side into a cylinder and seal it,

7. Using a knife or dental floss, break it in two. Split every half into four bits of similar size. In the end, you're expected to get 8 bits in one ball.

8. Move the slices to a 9-inch circular pan with oil. (Slice each cylinder into nine parts if a square pan is used. Or a 13 x 9-inch metal pan that contains 16 rolls.

9. For the leftover dough, repeat measures 5 through 8.

10. Cover with a kitchen towel and inexpensive prepare rolls. In a warm spot, let the rolls grow until they are not yet double in height.

11. Bake for 13 minutes or until the rolls are brownish on the edges in a preheated 350° F oven. A quick-read thermometer can read 190° F.

12. Leave the rolls to chill for almost 10 minutes in the pan. Switch rolls out on a refrigeration rack. It is possible that keeping rolls in the pan before they are cold results in soggy bottoms.

13. Create the icing until you take the rolls out.

14. Onto a microwave-safe, Pyrex quart measuring cup, put chocolate squares and butter. Microwave for two minutes, stirring through to melt the butter with chocolate uniformly on 50 percent strength.

15. Add the whisked milk sugar powder. Stir rapidly until the icing begins to glow and is smooth. To get the icing pourable, try adding more milk if necessary.

16. Use a spoon to glaze icing on over rolls.

Frosted Cinnamon Rolls

Preparation Time: 45 minutes |**Servings:** 21 rolls |**Difficulty: Easy**

Ingredients:

- Warm milk, one cup

- Water, (room temperature) a quarter cup

- Butter softened, a quarter cup

- One large egg

- Salt, one teaspoon

- Bread flour, four cups

- Instant vanilla pudding mix, a quarter cup

- Sugar, one tablespoon

- Active dry yeast, one tablespoon

Filling:

- Butter softened, a quarter cup

- Packed brown sugar, one cup

- The ground cinnamon, two teaspoons

Frosting:

- Cream cheese, softened, 4 ounces

- Butter softened, a quarter cup

- Confectioners' sugar, one and a half cups

- Milk, one and a half teaspoon

- Vanilla extract, half teaspoon

Instructions:

1. Place the first nine ingredients in the bread machine pan in order. Pick Dough Setup (check dough after 5 minutes of mixing; add one-two tablespoons of water or flour if needed).

2. Turn the dough onto a gently floured surface when the cycle is finished. Roll into a 17x10-inch, for a square. Using butter to spread, scatter with brown sugar and cinnamon. Roll up, beginning from a long hand, jellyroll style, pinch seam to seal. Split into 21 pieces.

3. In an oiled 13x9-inch, put 12 slices, cut side down. In a 9-inch square pan, baking tray, put nine rolls. Cover: cause to rise until doubled, around 45 minutes, in a warm place.

4. Bake for 20-25 minutes at 350°F or until golden brown. Cool for 10 minutes on wire racks.

5. Beat the frosting ingredients in a wide bowl until smooth.

6. Apply the frost on the baked rolls and enjoy.

Chocolate Chip Peanut Butter Banana Bread

Preparation Time: 3 hours 15 minutes |Servings: One loaf |Difficulty: Hard

Ingredients

- Three whole eggs

- Half cup of softened butter

- One and a half cups of mashed bananas (very ripe)

- One and a quarter cups of sugar

- Half cup of vegetable oil

- One and a half cups of all-purpose flour

- One teaspoon of salt

- Half cup of plain Greek yogurt

- One teaspoon of vanilla

- One cup of peanut butter and chocolate chips

- One teaspoon of baking soda

Instructions:

1. Add all ingredients, except chocolate chips and nuts, to the bread machine in the manufacturer's suggested order.

2. Select a batter bread cycle. Press the start button.

3. Add chocolate chips and nuts at the ingredient signal and take out the paddle.

4. Enjoy fresh bread.

Apple Kuchen

Preparation Time: 2 hours 10 minutes |Servings: 26 |Difficulty: Hard

Ingredients:

- Water, ½ cup

- Milk, a quarter cup

- Butter, ¾ cup

- Four eggs

- All-purpose flour, three cups

- Salt, half teaspoon

- Sugar, a quarter teaspoon

- Active Dry Yeast, one package

For the topping:

- Apples, two cups

- Pecans, (chopped) half cup

- Sugar, ⅓ cup

- Butter, (melted) a quarter cup

- Cinnamon, one teaspoon

- Lemon rind, (grated) one teaspoon

For the butter sauce:

- Half-and-Half cream, half cup

- Vanilla, one teaspoon

- Sugar, one cup

- Butter, half cup

Instructions:

1. In the order mentioned, put the ingredients in the pan. Set the dough/manual cycle range. Do not use the timer for gaps. Release the lid of the bread machine after 5 minutes of kneading. Scrape the rubber spatula on the bread tray's sides, transferring the soft flour to the kneading blade to blend properly. Do not add additional flour. Remove the butter when the cycle is complete.

2. Topping: Mix all the topping components in a medium dish.

3. Stir down the batter. Spread it in a 13x9-inch oiled cake tray. Topping Spoon over batter. Cover, stop for 10 minutes to rest. Bake in a preheated 350°F oven until golden brown for 45 to 50 minutes.

4. Prepare Butter Sauce: In a saucepan, butter, add sugar and half-and-a-half of milk. Heat to the boiling point, simmer until it thickens, stirring periodically. Put vanilla. Stir to blend.

5. Pour the sauce and the toppings over the bread and then serve.

English Muffin Bread

Preparation Time: 3 hours 40 minutes |Servings: One loaf |Difficulty: Hard

Ingredients:

- One cup of Lukewarm milk

- One teaspoon of vinegar

- Two tablespoons of butter

- 1/3 to a quarter cup of water

- One and a half teaspoons of salt

- Two and a quarter teaspoon of instant yeast

- Three and a half cups of all-purpose flour

- One and a half teaspoons of sugar

- Half teaspoon of baking powder

Instructions:

1. In the tin of the bread machine, add all ingredients. Use less water in a humid environment and more water in a dry or colder environment.

2. Select basic and light crust. Press the start button. Adjust dough consistency by adding more flour if too sticky and add water if too dry.

3. Serve fresh.

Cherry 'n Cheese Lattice Coffee Cake

Preparation Time: 1 hour |**Servings:** two cakes |**Difficulty: Hard**

Ingredients:

- Water, a quarter cup

- Two eggs

- Vanilla, one teaspoon

- Sour cream, half cup

- Butter, three tablespoons

- Sugar, three tablespoons

- Active Dry Yeast, one package

- Bread flour, three cups

- Salt, one and a half teaspoon

For the filling:

- Sugar, one tablespoon

- Salt, ⅛ teaspoon

- Cherry pie filling, one can

- Cream cheese, two packages

- One egg

For the icing

- Powdered sugar, one and a quarter cup

- Water, two tablespoons

Instructions:

1. Preheat oven to 350°F.

2. At room temperature, have liquid ingredients at 80°F and all other ingredients. In the order mentioned, put the dough ingredients in the bowl—dough/manual cycle selection. Verify the consistency of the dough after few minutes of kneading. The dough should be in a ball that is fluffy and tacky. Add water, half to one tablespoon at a time if it is dry and hard. Add one tablespoon of flour at a time if it is so sticky and messy. Remove the dough.

3. Cream the cream cheese, butter, egg, and salt together to prepare the filling. Punch the dough down and break it in two. Roll each half into a 12x17-inch rectangle on a lightly floured base. Spread half of the filling over the middle third of the dough lengthwise. Cover with half or so of the pie filling. (Save a few cherries after it is cooked from filling to decorate the coffee cake.) Cut one-inch-wide strips, two inches deep, on each long side. Fold strips at an angle around the filling, variously from side to side, beginning at one point. Place the coffee cake on a baking sheet with oil.

4. Cover; let rise, roughly 30 minutes, after gently contacting the side of the coffee cake. Bake for 30 to 35 minutes in a preheated oven. On a wire rack, cool.

Conclusion

Bread Machine is very simple and impressive, and it saves a lot of time. Perfect for unqualified cooks or limited-time cooks. Every other day, you can easily make fresh bread with no hustle. No more semi-stale supermarket bread that's been sitting for months in your freezer.

Some people might think it is sloppy to bake bread at home, and, ultimately, it's a tough operation. With a bread machine, though, baking bread is a breeze. You pick the desired choice and relax - within the bread maker, the rising, stirring, and baking phase takes place, which often allows it a no-mess process. You will appreciate the homemade bread that is freshly cooked.

Many bread makers usually have a timer feature that enables the baking period to be scheduled for a certain time. This feature is really useful in terms of flavor and consistency when you choose to get hot bread in the morning, or dinner and homemade bread still beats store-bought bread.

Let's face it, bread-making is a long and time-consuming process. It may be enjoyable to bake bread on the weekend, but when you come home after work during a workweek and still have to take care of the family, the possibility of finding a burst of energy to make fresh bread is small.

A bread machine is an option for you if you are the kind of person who needs fresh bread every day.

Especially if you like to wake up to the scent of fresh bread filling the house in the morning, many bread machines have a timer that you can set in the middle of the night, and you can wake up in the morning to the scent of fresh bread with only one click of a button.

CPSIA information can be obtained
at www.ICGtesting.com
Printed in the USA
LVHW080336300621
691543LV00003B/259

9 781802 169508